Table Of Contents

Introduction

The importance of organic beauty

The importance of organic beauty is something that cannot be overstated. As we become more aware of the impact our choices have on the environment and our health, it's becoming increasingly clear that choosing organic beauty products is one of the best things we can do for ourselves and the planet.

For starters, organic beauty products are free of harmful chemicals and toxins that can be found in conventional beauty products. These chemicals can be absorbed into our skin and can cause a variety of health problems, such as hormonal imbalances and allergies. By choosing organic beauty products, we can avoid these risks and ensure that we are using products that are safe and healthy for us.

Organic beauty products are also better for the environment. The ingredients used in these products are grown without the use of pesticides and other harmful chemicals that can pollute our air and water. Organic farming practices are also better for the soil, promoting biodiversity and preserving natural habitats.

In addition to being better for our health and the environment, organic beauty products can also be more effective than their conventional counterparts. Organic ingredients are often more nutrient-dense and can provide more benefits to our skin and hair.

Natural ingredients like aloe vera, coconut oil, and shea butter can hydrate and nourish our skin, while essential oils can provide a variety of therapeutic benefits.

Finally, choosing organic beauty products can be a great way to support small businesses and local economies. Many organic beauty brands are small and independently owned, and by choosing their products, we can help to support these businesses and the communities they serve.

Overall, the importance of organic beauty cannot be overstated. By choosing organic beauty products, we can protect our health, the environment, and support small businesses. So the next time you're in the market for new beauty products, consider going organic – your body and the planet will thank you.

Why organic beauty is important for 30-year-olds

As a 30-year-old, your skin may not be as resilient as it once was. Environmental factors, lifestyle choices, and hormonal changes can all impact the health and appearance of your skin. That's why it's important to adopt an organic beauty routine that caters to your unique needs.

Organic beauty products are made with natural ingredients that are grown without the use of pesticides, synthetic fertilizers, or genetically modified organisms (GMOs). They are free from harsh chemicals that can strip your skin of its natural oils and cause irritation. Instead, they are gentle and nourishing, delivering the nutrients your skin needs to stay healthy and radiant.

One of the main benefits of organic beauty products is that they are better for the environment. Traditional beauty products often contain chemicals that can be harmful to the planet, contaminating the air, water, and soil. Organic products, on the other hand, are made with sustainable and eco-friendly practices that minimize their impact on the environment.

In addition to being better for you and the planet, organic beauty products are also more ethical. Many brands are committed to using fair trade ingredients and supporting local communities. They are often cruelty-free, meaning they don't test on animals, and vegan, meaning they don't contain any animal-derived ingredients.

If you're a young mom, organic beauty products are especially important for your family's health and wellbeing. Children are more vulnerable to the harmful effects of chemicals, so it's important to choose products that are safe and gentle. Organic skincare and natural makeup are great options for kids, as they are less likely to cause irritation or allergic reactions.

Overall, organic beauty is an essential part of any 30-year-old's self-care routine. By choosing natural, sustainable, and ethical products, you can enhance your beauty and protect your health and the planet. So why not give it a try and see the difference for yourself?

Overview of the book

Organic Beauty on a Budget: Tips and Tricks for 30 Year Olds is a comprehensive guide that offers practical and easy-to-follow advice on how to achieve beautiful, healthy, and glowing skin without breaking the bank. This book is designed for young adults, 30 year olds, and young moms who are interested in organic and natural beauty products but are concerned about the high cost of these products.

The book covers a wide range of topics related to organic beauty, including the benefits of organic and natural beauty products, how to read labels and understand ingredients, how to choose the right products for your skin type, and how to create a simple and effective beauty routine.

One of the key features of this book is its focus on budget-friendly organic beauty solutions. The author provides many tips and tricks for finding affordable organic and natural beauty products, as well as DIY recipes for making your own beauty products at home. You will learn how to make your own face masks, body scrubs, and hair treatments using ingredients that are easy to find and inexpensive.

In addition to providing practical advice on organic beauty, this book also addresses some of the common misconceptions about organic and natural beauty products. The author debunks the myth that organic and natural products are less effective than their synthetic counterparts and explains why organic and natural products are often better for your skin and overall health.

Overall, Organic Beauty on a Budget: Tips and Tricks for 30 Year Olds is an essential guide for anyone who wants to achieve beautiful, healthy, and glowing skin without spending a fortune on expensive beauty products. Whether you are a young adult, 30 year old, or young mom, this book will provide you with the knowledge and tools you need to make informed decisions about your beauty routine and achieve the radiant and healthy skin you deserve. If you are interested in organic beauty product website, organic skincare, natural makeup, or vegan beauty products, this book is a must-read!

The Basics of Organic Skincare

Understanding your skin type

Understanding Your Skin Type

One of the most important steps in achieving beautiful and healthy skin is understanding your skin type. Knowing your skin type will help you choose the right products and create a skincare routine that works for you.

There are four main skin types: oily, dry, combination, and sensitive. Here's a breakdown of each:

Oily Skin – If you have oily skin, your skin tends to produce more oil than necessary, which can lead to clogged pores and breakouts. Your skin may also appear shiny and feel greasy to the touch.

Dry Skin – On the other hand, if you have dry skin, your skin may feel tight and flaky. You may also experience redness and irritation.

Combination Skin – Combination skin is a mix of both oily and dry skin. Your T-zone (forehead, nose, and chin) may be oily, while the rest of your face may be dry.

Sensitive Skin – Sensitive skin is easily irritated and may react to certain products or ingredients. You may experience redness, itching, and dryness.

It's important to note that your skin type can change over time depending on factors such as age, hormones, and weather conditions. So, it's important to reassess your skin type periodically to make sure you're using the right products.

Once you've identified your skin type, you can start looking for products that cater to your specific needs. For example, if you have oily skin, look for products that contain salicylic acid or benzoyl peroxide to help control oil and prevent breakouts. If you have dry skin, look for products that contain hyaluronic acid or ceramides to help hydrate and moisturize your skin.

Remember, there's no one-size-fits-all when it comes to skincare. What works for one person may not work for another. So, it's important to experiment with different products and find what works best for you.

In conclusion, understanding your skin type is the first step in achieving beautiful and healthy skin. Take the time to assess your skin type and choose products that cater to your specific needs. With a little bit of effort and experimentation, you can create a skincare routine that works for you and fits your budget.

The benefits of organic skincare

The benefits of organic skincare are numerous and cannot be overlooked. With the increasing awareness about the harmful effects of chemicals in beauty products, more and more people are turning towards organic skincare. In this subchapter, we will discuss some of the benefits of organic skincare.

Firstly, organic skincare products are made from natural ingredients that are free from harmful chemicals. These products are gentle on the skin and do not cause any adverse reactions. Unlike conventional skincare products, organic skincare products do not contain parabens, sulfates, or phthalates, which are known to cause skin irritation, allergies, and even cancer.

Secondly, organic skincare products are rich in antioxidants, vitamins, and minerals that nourish the skin. These ingredients help to repair damaged skin cells and promote the growth of new ones. They also help to reduce the appearance of fine lines and wrinkles, making the skin look younger and healthier.

Thirdly, organic skincare products are eco-friendly and sustainable. They are made from natural ingredients that are grown without the use of harmful pesticides and fertilizers. This means that they do not harm the environment and are safe to use.

Fourthly, organic skincare products are cruelty-free and vegan. They are not tested on animals and do not contain any animal-derived ingredients. This makes them a great choice for those who are conscious of animal welfare and want to support ethical and sustainable practices.

In conclusion, organic skincare products offer numerous benefits that cannot be overlooked. They are gentle on the skin, rich in antioxidants and other beneficial ingredients, eco-friendly and sustainable, and cruelty-free and vegan. If you are looking for a way to take care of your skin in a natural and healthy way, then organic skincare products are the way to go.

Ingredients to avoid in conventional skincare products

When we go shopping for skincare products, we are often overwhelmed by the vast array of options available on the shelves. However, not all of these products are created equal, and some may contain harmful ingredients that can have long-term effects on our skin and overall health. In this subchapter, we will discuss some of the ingredients to avoid in conventional skincare products and why it's important to choose organic and natural alternatives.

Parabens: Parabens are a group of synthetic preservatives commonly used in skincare products to extend their shelf life. However, they have been linked to hormonal imbalances, breast cancer, and other health issues. Look out for ingredients such as methylparaben, ethylparaben, propylparaben, and butylparaben on the label.

Phthalates: Phthalates are plasticizers that are added to skincare products to make them more flexible and pliable. They are often used in fragrances, lotions, and nail polishes. However, they can disrupt the endocrine system and cause developmental defects, reproductive issues, and asthma. Avoid ingredients such as dibutyl phthalate, diethyl phthalate, and dimethyl phthalate.

Sulfates: Sulfates are surfactants that are added to skincare products to create lather and foam. They can strip the skin of its natural oils and cause irritation, dryness, and even acne. Avoid ingredients such as sodium lauryl sulfate (SLS) and sodium laureth sulfate (SLES).

Artificial fragrances: Artificial fragrances are often added to skincare products to enhance their scent. However, they can contain dozens of harmful chemicals that can cause allergies, skin irritation, and even cancer. Look out for ingredients such as parfum, fragrance, and perfume on the label.

In conclusion, it's crucial to read the labels of skincare products and avoid ingredients that can harm our skin and health. By choosing organic and natural alternatives, we can protect our skin and the environment while still enjoying the benefits of effective skincare.

DIY organic skincare recipes

DIY Organic Skincare Recipes

Creating your own organic skincare products at home can be a fun and cost-effective way to achieve healthy, glowing skin. By using natural ingredients, you can avoid harsh chemicals and preservatives that can be found in many store-bought products. Here are some simple recipes to get you started:

1. Coconut oil and sugar scrub: Mix together equal parts coconut oil and sugar to create a gentle exfoliating scrub. Massage onto damp skin in circular motions, then rinse off with warm water. This will leave your skin feeling soft and moisturized.

2. Avocado and honey face mask: Mash together half an avocado and two tablespoons of honey to create a nourishing face mask. Apply to clean skin and leave on for 15-20 minutes before rinsing off with warm water. This mask is packed with antioxidants and vitamins that will leave your skin looking and feeling refreshed.

3. Green tea and aloe vera toner: Brew a cup of green tea and let it cool. Mix in a tablespoon of aloe vera gel and pour into a spray bottle. Spritz onto your face after cleansing to help soothe and hydrate your skin.

4. Oatmeal and honey facial cleanser: Mix together equal parts ground oatmeal and honey to create a gentle cleanser. Massage onto damp skin in circular motions, then rinse off with warm water. This will help remove dirt and impurities while also moisturizing your skin.

5. Rosewater and witch hazel toner: Mix together equal parts rosewater and witch hazel to create a refreshing toner. Apply to clean skin with a cotton pad to help balance and tone your skin.

These are just a few examples of the many DIY organic skincare recipes you can create at home. Not only are these recipes all-natural and effective, but they are also affordable and easy to make. By incorporating these recipes into your skincare routine, you can achieve healthy, glowing skin without breaking the bank.

Building a Natural Makeup Collection

The importance of natural makeup

The Importance of Natural Makeup

When it comes to makeup, most people focus on the look they want to achieve. However, it is important to pay attention to the products you use, especially if you want to maintain your skin's health. Natural makeup, also known as organic makeup, is an excellent way to achieve the look you want without compromising your skin's health. Here are some reasons why natural makeup is essential for your beauty routine.

1. Natural makeup is gentler on your skin

Many traditional makeup products contain harsh chemicals, fragrances, and synthetic ingredients that can irritate the skin. Natural makeup, on the other hand, is made from plant-based ingredients that are gentle and safe for all skin types. It also contains antioxidants and vitamins that can help nourish and protect your skin.

2. Natural makeup is better for the environment

Traditional makeup products are often packaged in non-recyclable plastics and contain ingredients that are harmful to the environment. Natural makeup, on the other hand, is made from sustainable and biodegradable ingredients that are better for the planet.

3. Natural makeup is cruelty-free

Most natural makeup products are made without animal testing, which means they are cruelty-free. If you are a vegan or animal lover, this is an important consideration when choosing makeup products.

4. Natural makeup is long-lasting

Natural makeup products are made with high-quality ingredients that are designed to last longer than traditional makeup products. This means that you can achieve the same look with fewer touch-ups throughout the day.

5. Natural makeup is versatile

Natural makeup products come in a wide range of shades and textures, making it easy to find the perfect product for your skin type and color. Whether you want a natural, everyday look or a dramatic, nighttime look, there is a natural makeup product that will meet your needs.

In conclusion, natural makeup is an essential part of any beauty routine. It is gentle on the skin, better for the environment, cruelty-free, long-lasting, and versatile. If you want to maintain healthy, beautiful skin, consider switching to natural makeup products.

Ingredients to avoid in conventional makeup products

When it comes to makeup, we all want products that make us look and feel good. However, not all makeup products are created equal. Many conventional makeup products contain harmful ingredients that can cause long-term damage to our skin and overall health. As young adults, 30-year-olds, and young moms, it is important to be mindful of the ingredients in the makeup products we use, as they can have a significant impact on our health and wellbeing.

Here are some of the ingredients to avoid in conventional makeup products:

1. Parabens: Parabens are a type of preservative used in many makeup products. They have been linked to hormone disruption and breast cancer. Look for products labeled "paraben-free."

2. Phthalates: Phthalates are chemicals used to make plastics more flexible. They are often found in fragrances and have been linked to reproductive problems and birth defects.

3. Synthetic fragrances: Synthetic fragrances can contain hundreds of chemicals, many of which are toxic. Look for products with natural fragrances or no fragrance at all.

4. Formaldehyde: Formaldehyde is a carcinogen and can cause skin irritation and allergies. It is often found in nail polish and hair products.

5. Lead: Lead is a toxic metal that can accumulate in the body over time. It is often found in lipsticks and can cause neurological damage.

6. Petroleum-based ingredients: Petroleum-based ingredients, such as mineral oil and petrolatum, can clog pores and cause acne. They are also a non-renewable resource.

7. Talc: Talc is a mineral that is often found in powder makeup products. It has been linked to ovarian cancer and lung problems.

By avoiding these ingredients, you can ensure that the makeup products you use are safe and healthy for your skin. Look for organic, natural, and vegan beauty products that are free from harmful chemicals. Your skin and overall health will thank you for it.

Tips for finding natural makeup products

Tips for finding natural makeup products

In today's world, the importance of using organic and natural products has been recognized by many people. When it comes to makeup, natural and organic products are becoming increasingly popular as they not only provide a flawless and beautiful look but also offer various skin benefits. However, finding the right natural makeup products can be challenging, especially when you are on a budget. Here are some tips to help you find the best natural makeup products:

1. Read the ingredient list

The first and most crucial step in finding natural makeup products is to read the ingredient list. Always check the label for ingredients that are chemical-free, organic, and natural. Avoid products that contain harmful chemicals like parabens, phthalates, and synthetic fragrances.

2. Check for certifications

When looking for natural makeup products, check for certifications like USDA organic, Non-GMO Project Verified, and Leaping Bunny Certified. These certifications ensure that the product is made from safe, natural, and cruelty-free ingredients.

3. Look for reviews

Before purchasing any natural makeup product, take the time to read reviews from other customers. Reading reviews will give you an idea of the product's effectiveness, quality, and overall performance.

4. Choose multi-purpose products

Another way to save money on natural makeup products is to choose multi-purpose products. For example, a natural lip and cheek tint can be used as a lip color, blush, and even eyeshadow.

5. Buy in bulk

Buying natural makeup products in bulk can save you money in the long run. Many natural makeup brands offer discounts on bulk purchases. Moreover, buying in bulk also reduces packaging waste, making it an eco-friendly option.

In conclusion, finding natural makeup products requires some research and effort. Don't be afraid to try different brands and products until you find the right one for you. By following these tips, you can find affordable, natural, and high-quality makeup products that suit your needs and budget.

DIY natural makeup recipes

DIY Natural Makeup Recipes

Makeup is an essential part of our daily routine, but not all of us are aware of the harmful chemicals used in commercial makeup products. The chemicals used in these products can harm our skin and even lead to serious health issues. But, don't worry, there is a solution – DIY natural makeup recipes.

Making your own natural makeup is not only safe and healthy for your skin, but it is also cost-effective and eco-friendly. In this section, we will share some easy and effective DIY natural makeup recipes that you can try at home.

1. Lip Balm

This lip balm recipe is super easy to make and will leave your lips feeling soft and moisturized. You will need:

- 1 tablespoon beeswax
- 1 tablespoon shea butter
- 1 tablespoon coconut oil
- 1-2 drops of essential oil (optional)

Melt the beeswax, shea butter, and coconut oil in a double boiler. Once melted, remove from heat and add essential oil (if using). Pour into a lip balm container and let it cool.

2. Mascara

Commercial mascaras often contain harmful chemicals that can irritate your eyes. This natural mascara recipe is gentle on your eyes, and it will give you longer and thicker lashes. You will need:

- 1 teaspoon activated charcoal
- 1 teaspoon coconut oil
- 1 teaspoon aloe vera gel

Mix all the ingredients in a small bowl until you get a smooth paste. Transfer the mixture to an old mascara tube or any small container and use it as you would use regular mascara.

3. Blush

This DIY blush recipe is perfect for adding a natural flush to your cheeks. You will need:

- 1 tablespoon arrowroot powder
- 1-2 drops of beetroot juice
- 1-2 drops of essential oil (optional)

Mix the arrowroot powder, beetroot juice, and essential oil (if using) in a small bowl until you get a smooth consistency. Apply it to your cheeks with a blush brush.

In conclusion, making your own natural makeup is an excellent alternative to commercial makeup products. These DIY natural makeup recipes are easy to make and will leave your skin feeling healthy and beautiful. Give them a try and see the difference for yourself.

Vegan Beauty Products

The benefits of vegan beauty products

The beauty industry has been evolving over the years, and one of the latest trends that have taken the market by storm is vegan beauty products. These products are free from animal-derived ingredients and have a host of benefits for your skin, hair, and overall health. In this subchapter, we will explore the benefits of vegan beauty products and why they are an excellent choice for Young Adults, 30 year olds, and Young Moms who are looking for organic beauty products.

Firstly, vegan beauty products are gentle on your skin. They are free from harsh chemicals, preservatives, and synthetic fragrances that can irritate your skin. Instead, they use natural ingredients that are rich in vitamins, minerals, and antioxidants that nourish your skin. This means that vegan beauty products are ideal for people with sensitive skin or those who are prone to allergies.

Secondly, vegan beauty products are environmentally friendly. They do not involve any animal testing or animal cruelty, which means that you can use them with a clear conscience. Moreover, vegan beauty products are made using sustainable and eco-friendly ingredients that do not harm the environment. By using vegan beauty products, you are contributing to a more sustainable future.

Thirdly, vegan beauty products are effective. Contrary to popular belief, vegan beauty products are not just a fad. They are formulated using natural ingredients that are backed by science and have been proven to work. For instance, plant-based oils such as coconut oil, avocado oil, and jojoba oil are excellent for hydrating and moisturizing your skin. Similarly, natural ingredients such as aloe vera, chamomile, and lavender have anti-inflammatory properties that soothe and calm your skin.

In conclusion, vegan beauty products are an excellent choice for anyone looking for organic beauty products. They are gentle on your skin, environmentally friendly, and effective. Whether you are looking for organic skincare, natural makeup, or vegan beauty products, there is something for everyone in the world of vegan beauty.

Ingredients to avoid in non-vegan beauty products

When it comes to beauty products, it's important to not only consider the benefits they can bring to your skin, but also the ingredients they contain. Unfortunately, many non-vegan beauty products include ingredients that can be harmful to both your health and the environment.

Here are some of the most common ingredients to avoid in non-vegan beauty products:

1. Parabens: These are synthetic preservatives that are often used in cosmetics and skincare products to prevent the growth of bacteria and mold. However, they have been linked to hormone disruption and breast cancer.

2. Phthalates: These are a group of chemicals that are used to make plastics more flexible and durable. They are often found in fragrances and have been linked to reproductive and developmental problems.

3. Formaldehyde: This is a preservative that is used in a variety of beauty products, including nail polish and hair treatments. It has been linked to cancer and respiratory problems.

4. Sodium lauryl sulfate (SLS): This is a foaming agent that is often used in shampoos and body washes. It can be irritating to the skin and eyes, and has been linked to hormone disruption.

5. Animal-derived ingredients: Many non-vegan beauty products contain ingredients that are derived from animals, such as lanolin (from sheep's wool), collagen (from animal bones and skin), and carmine (a red pigment made from crushed beetles). Not only are these ingredients not vegan-friendly, but they can also be harmful to the environment.

By avoiding these ingredients in your beauty products, you can help protect both your health and the environment. Look for products that are vegan, organic, and free from harmful chemicals. Your skin (and the planet) will thank you!

Tips for finding vegan beauty products

Tips for Finding Vegan Beauty Products

If you're looking for vegan beauty products, you're in luck! There are plenty of options out there, but it can be overwhelming to know where to start. Here are some tips for finding the best vegan beauty products for you:

1. Look for the vegan label

One of the easiest ways to find vegan beauty products is to look for products with the vegan label. This means that the product is certified vegan and does not contain any animal products or byproducts. This label is typically found on the packaging or on the company's website.

2. Research the company's animal testing policy

Just because a product is vegan doesn't necessarily mean that it's cruelty-free. Make sure to research the company's animal testing policy to ensure that they do not test their products on animals. Look for products that are certified cruelty-free by organizations such as PETA or Leaping Bunny.

3. Check the ingredients list

While a product may be labeled as vegan, it's still important to check the ingredients list to ensure that it doesn't contain any animal-derived ingredients. Look out for ingredients such as beeswax, lanolin, and carmine, which are commonly found in beauty products.

4. Read reviews

Reading reviews from other customers can give you an idea of how well a vegan beauty product works. Look for reviews from people with similar skin types or concerns to yours to get the most accurate information.

5. Consider the price

Vegan beauty products can range in price from affordable to high-end. While it's important to invest in quality skincare and makeup, make sure to consider your budget when shopping for vegan beauty products.

By following these tips, you can find the best vegan beauty products for your skincare and makeup routine. Remember to always do your research and read the ingredients list to ensure that the products you're using are truly vegan and cruelty-free.

DIY vegan beauty product recipes

DIY vegan beauty product recipes are becoming a popular trend for those who want to use natural and organic ingredients on their skin. These recipes are not only affordable but also easy to make and customize based on personal preferences. In this subchapter, we will discuss some DIY vegan beauty product recipes that are perfect for young adults, 30 year olds, and young moms who are interested in organic beauty products.

The first recipe is for a homemade facial cleanser that uses just three ingredients: coconut oil, castile soap, and essential oils. To make this cleanser, simply mix 1/4 cup of melted coconut oil with 1/4 cup of castile soap and a few drops of your favorite essential oil. This cleanser is gentle on the skin and effective at removing dirt and makeup.

Next, we have a recipe for a vegan lip balm that is perfect for dry, chapped lips. To make this lip balm, you will need coconut oil, shea butter, and candelilla wax. Simply melt together one tablespoon of coconut oil, one tablespoon of shea butter, and one tablespoon of candelilla wax. Once melted, pour into a small container and let it cool. This lip balm is moisturizing and nourishing for the lips.

For those who want a natural alternative to store-bought deodorant, we have a recipe for a vegan deodorant that uses baking soda, arrowroot powder, coconut oil, and essential oils. Simply mix together 1/4 cup of baking soda, 1/4 cup of arrowroot powder, and 1/4 cup of melted coconut oil. Add a few drops of your favorite essential oil and mix well. This deodorant is effective at controlling odor and keeping you feeling fresh all day long.

Lastly, we have a recipe for a homemade body scrub that uses sugar, coconut oil, and essential oils. Mix together one cup of sugar and 1/2 cup of melted coconut oil. Add a few drops of your favorite essential oil and mix well. This body scrub is perfect for exfoliating and moisturizing the skin.

In conclusion, DIY vegan beauty product recipes are a great way to incorporate natural and organic ingredients into your skincare routine. These recipes are affordable, easy to make, and customizable to fit your personal preferences. By using these recipes, you can have healthy, glowing skin without breaking the bank.

Organic Beauty on a Budget

Tips for saving money on organic beauty products

Organic beauty products are a great way to take care of your skin and hair without exposing yourself to harmful chemicals. However, they can also be expensive, which can be a deterrent for many people who are on a budget. Fortunately, there are several ways to save money on organic beauty products without compromising on quality. Here are some tips that can help you save money while still enjoying the benefits of organic beauty products.

1. Look for sales and discounts: Many organic beauty product websites offer regular sales and discounts on their products. Keep an eye out for these offers and stock up on your favorite products when they are on sale.

2. Buy in bulk: Buying organic beauty products in bulk can help you save money in the long run. Look for products that have a longer shelf life and buy them in larger quantities.

3. Make your own products: Making your own organic beauty products at home can be a fun and cost-effective way to care for your skin and hair. You can find many recipes for DIY organic beauty products online, and most of the ingredients you need can be found in your kitchen.

4. Choose multi-purpose products: Look for organic beauty products that can be used for multiple purposes. For example, a face oil can also be used as a body moisturizer, or a lip balm can double as a cuticle cream.

5. Use samples and trial sizes: Many organic beauty product websites offer samples and trial sizes of their products. This can be a great way to try out new products without committing to a full-size purchase.

6. Opt for simple products: Some organic beauty products contain a long list of ingredients, which can drive up the price. Look for products that have simple and natural ingredients, as they are often less expensive.

7. Join loyalty programs: Many organic beauty product websites offer loyalty programs that give you points for your purchases. These points can be redeemed for discounts on future purchases.

By following these tips, you can save money on organic beauty products without sacrificing quality. Whether you are a young adult, a young mom, or someone who is passionate about organic skincare, natural makeup, or vegan beauty products, these tips can help you build a budget-friendly organic beauty routine that works for you.

Making the most of your beauty budget

When it comes to beauty, it's easy to get caught up in all the hype surrounding the latest and greatest products. But with so many options out there, it can be overwhelming to know where to start and what to invest in. That's why it's important to have a budget in mind and make the most of it by focusing on the essentials.

First, prioritize your skincare routine. A good cleanser, moisturizer, and sunscreen are must-haves for healthy, glowing skin. Look for organic and natural options that are free of harsh chemicals and synthetic fragrances. These products may cost a bit more upfront, but they often last longer and are better for your skin in the long run.

Next, consider investing in a few multi-purpose products that can save you time and money. For example, a tinted moisturizer with SPF can serve as a moisturizer, sunscreen, and light coverage all in one. A versatile lip and cheek tint can add a pop of color to your lips and cheeks, but also double as an eyeshadow. Look for products that are vegan and cruelty-free to align with your values.

When it comes to makeup, focus on quality over quantity. A few high-quality products can make all the difference in your overall look. Choose a foundation or concealer that matches your skin tone perfectly and lasts throughout the day. Invest in a good set of brushes that can be used for multiple products, and consider splurging on a signature lipstick shade that makes you feel confident and beautiful.

Lastly, don't forget about the power of self-care. Taking care of your mental and emotional well-being can do wonders for your overall beauty. Set aside time for a relaxing bath with essential oils, practice mindfulness meditation, or treat yourself to a massage or facial. These self-care practices can help reduce stress and promote a healthy, radiant glow.

In conclusion, making the most of your beauty budget is about focusing on the essentials, investing in multi-purpose products, choosing quality over quantity, and prioritizing self-care. By following these tips, you can achieve a natural, organic beauty routine that aligns with your values and makes you feel confident and beautiful.

DIY beauty product recipes for a fraction of the cost

DIY Beauty Product Recipes for a Fraction of the Cost

If you're on a budget but still want to look and feel your best, then DIY beauty product recipes are the way to go. By making your own products at home, you can save a ton of money while still getting the same benefits as expensive store-bought products. Here are some easy and affordable recipes for natural and organic beauty products that you can make at home.

1. Coconut oil hair mask - Coconut oil is a great natural moisturizer for your hair. Simply warm up some coconut oil and

apply it to your hair, focusing on the ends. Leave it on for at least 30 minutes before washing it out with shampoo.

2. Coffee body scrub - Coffee grounds are a great natural exfoliator for your skin. Mix together some coffee grounds, coconut oil, and brown sugar to make a scrub that will leave your skin soft and smooth.

3. Green tea toner - Green tea is packed with antioxidants that are great for your skin. Steep some green tea and let it cool, then use it as a toner by applying it to your face with a cotton pad.

4. Avocado face mask - Avocado is a great source of healthy fats that are beneficial for your skin. Mash up an avocado and mix it with some honey and lemon juice to make a hydrating face mask.

5. Lip balm - Making your own lip balm is easy and affordable. Melt together some coconut oil, beeswax, and your favorite essential oils, then pour the mixture into small containers.

By making your own beauty products at home, you can save money and avoid harmful chemicals that are often found in store-bought products. These DIY recipes are simple and effective, and they're perfect for anyone who wants to look and feel their best without breaking the bank.

Maintaining Healthy Skin

The link between diet and healthy skin

The link between diet and healthy skin is undeniable. What you eat reflects on your skin, and it is important to understand the connection between the two.

If you want to have healthy, glowing skin, you need to nourish it from within. A balanced diet that includes plenty of fruits, vegetables, and healthy fats can help you achieve just that. Foods that are rich in antioxidants, vitamins, and minerals help protect your skin cells from damage and aging.

One of the most important nutrients for healthy skin is collagen. Collagen is a protein that gives your skin its structure and elasticity. As you age, your body produces less collagen, which can lead to wrinkles, sagging, and dull skin. However, you can boost your collagen production by eating foods that are rich in vitamin C, such as citrus fruits, berries, and leafy greens.

Another key nutrient for healthy skin is omega-3 fatty acids. These healthy fats help keep your skin hydrated and supple, and also have anti-inflammatory properties. You can find omega-3s in fatty fish, such as salmon and mackerel, as well as in nuts and seeds.

On the other hand, there are certain foods that can be harmful to your skin. Processed foods, sugary drinks, and alcohol can all contribute to inflammation, which can lead to acne, redness, and premature aging. Additionally, dairy products have been linked to acne, so it may be worth cutting back on milk, cheese, and yogurt if you struggle with breakouts.

In conclusion, if you want to have healthy, beautiful skin, it's important to pay attention to what you eat. A diet that is rich in fruits, vegetables, healthy fats, and lean protein can help you achieve the glowing skin you desire. So next time you're at the grocery store, think about how your food choices will affect your skin, and choose wisely.

Nutrients that promote healthy skin

Nutrients that promote healthy skin

Your skin is the largest organ in your body, and it requires proper nourishment to maintain its health and beauty. While many people focus on external skincare routines, it's important to remember that what you put inside your body can be just as important. Here are some of the nutrients that promote healthy skin:

1. Vitamin C: This is a powerful antioxidant that helps to protect your skin from damage caused by free radicals. It also helps to boost collagen production, which is essential for maintaining skin elasticity and reducing the appearance of fine lines and wrinkles.

Foods that are rich in vitamin C include citrus fruits, strawberries, kiwi, and bell peppers.

2. Vitamin E: Another antioxidant, vitamin E helps to protect your skin from damage caused by the sun and other environmental factors. It also helps to soothe and hydrate dry or irritated skin. Foods that are rich in vitamin E include nuts, seeds, avocados, and leafy greens.

3. Omega-3 fatty acids: These healthy fats help to keep your skin supple and hydrated. They also have anti-inflammatory properties that can help to reduce redness and irritation. Foods that are rich in omega-3s include fatty fish like salmon, nuts and seeds, and flaxseed oil.

4. Zinc: This mineral is essential for maintaining healthy skin, as it helps to regulate oil production and heal wounds. It also has anti-inflammatory properties that can help to reduce acne and other skin irritations. Foods that are rich in zinc include oysters, beef, pumpkin seeds, and chickpeas.

5. Biotin: This B vitamin is essential for healthy skin, hair, and nails. It helps to strengthen the skin barrier and prevent dryness and flakiness. Foods that are rich in biotin include eggs, almonds, sweet potatoes, and spinach.

Incorporating these nutrients into your diet can help to promote healthy, glowing skin from the inside out. Remember to also use high-quality organic beauty products on your skin to further enhance its health and appearance.

Tips for maintaining healthy skin at home

Maintaining healthy skin at home is crucial not only for your appearance but for your overall well-being. Our skin is the largest organ in the body, and taking care of it is essential. With the abundance of beauty products available on the market, it can be overwhelming to choose the right ones. However, with these tips, you can maintain healthy skin without breaking the bank.

1. Cleanse regularly

Cleansing your skin is the first step to maintaining healthy skin. It removes dirt, oil, and makeup from the skin, preventing clogged pores that can lead to breakouts. Choose a gentle cleanser that suits your skin type and cleanse your face twice a day, in the morning and at night.

2. Exfoliate weekly

Exfoliating removes dead skin cells, revealing a brighter complexion. It also helps to unclog pores, allowing your skin to absorb skincare products better. Choose a natural exfoliator that suits your skin type and exfoliate once a week.

3. Moisturize daily

Moisturizing your skin keeps it hydrated and prevents dryness, flakiness, and wrinkles. Choose a moisturizer that suits your skin type and apply it daily, in the morning and at night.

4. Use sunscreen

Sunscreen protects your skin from the harmful UV rays of the sun, preventing premature aging and skin cancer. Choose a sunscreen with an SPF of at least 30 and apply it daily, even on cloudy days.

5. Stay hydrated

Drinking plenty of water keeps your skin hydrated from the inside out. Aim for at least eight glasses of water a day to maintain healthy skin.

6. Eat a healthy diet

Eating a diet rich in fruits, vegetables, and whole grains provides your skin with the nutrients it needs to maintain its health. Avoid processed foods, sugary drinks, and alcohol, which can damage your skin.

7. Get enough sleep

Getting enough sleep is essential for maintaining healthy skin. Lack of sleep can lead to dark circles, puffiness, and dull skin. Aim for at least seven to eight hours of sleep every night.

Maintaining healthy skin at home doesn't have to be expensive. By following these tips, you can achieve healthy, glowing skin without breaking the bank. Remember to choose organic, natural, and vegan beauty products for the best results.

Natural remedies for common skin problems

Natural remedies for common skin problems

Taking care of your skin is essential, and sometimes, the best way to do it is by using natural remedies. Here are some organic skincare tips and tricks for young adults, 30 year olds, and young moms to help you address common skin problems effectively.

Acne

Acne is a common skin problem that affects many young adults. To treat acne naturally, you can use tea tree oil, which has antiseptic and anti-inflammatory properties. Dilute a few drops of tea tree oil in water and apply it to your face using a cotton ball. You can also use aloe vera gel, which has antibacterial and anti-inflammatory properties. Apply aloe vera gel to your face and leave it for 20 minutes before rinsing it off with water.

Dry skin

Dry skin can be itchy and uncomfortable, but you can treat it naturally using coconut oil. Coconut oil is rich in fatty acids that help to moisturize and nourish the skin. Apply coconut oil to your skin and massage it gently until it is absorbed. You can also use honey, which has humectant properties that help to retain moisture in the skin. Apply honey to your face and leave it for 15 minutes before rinsing it off with water.

Dark circles

Dark circles under the eyes can make you look tired and older than you are. To treat dark circles naturally, you can use cucumber slices, which have a cooling effect and contain antioxidants that help to reduce inflammation. Place cucumber slices on your eyes and leave them for 10-15 minutes. You can also use green tea bags, which contain caffeine and antioxidants that help to reduce puffiness and inflammation. Place green tea bags on your eyes and leave them for 10-15 minutes.

In conclusion, natural remedies can be effective in treating common skin problems. These organic skincare tips and tricks are suitable for those who are looking for natural makeup and vegan beauty products. By using these remedies, you can take care of your skin without breaking the bank.

Organic Beauty for Young Moms

The importance of organic beauty for moms

As a young mom, you're always on the go. Whether you're tending to your little ones or working, it's essential to take care of yourself. One of the best ways to do that is by using organic beauty products.

Organic beauty products are made from natural ingredients that are free from harmful chemicals. These products not only nourish your skin but also offer a host of other benefits. Here's why organic beauty is essential for young moms.

1. Safe for you and your baby

Conventional beauty products contain chemicals that can be harmful to you and your baby. Organic beauty products are made from natural ingredients that are free from toxins, making them safe for you and your baby.

2. Nourishes your skin

As a young mom, you're always on the go, and your skin takes a beating. Organic beauty products are packed with nutrients that nourish your skin, leaving it soft and supple.

3. Protects the environment

Conventional beauty products contain ingredients that are harmful to the environment. Organic beauty products are made from natural ingredients that are sustainable and eco-friendly.

4. Cruelty-free

Many conventional beauty products are tested on animals, which is cruel and unnecessary. Organic beauty products are cruelty-free, meaning they're not tested on animals.

5. Affordable

Contrary to popular belief, organic beauty products are affordable. You don't have to break the bank to take care of your skin. There are many organic beauty products that are budget-friendly.

In conclusion, organic beauty is essential for young moms. It's safe, nourishing, eco-friendly, cruelty-free, and affordable. If you're looking for organic beauty products, check out our website for a range of natural makeup, vegan beauty products, and organic skincare.

Simple beauty routines for busy moms

Simple beauty routines for busy moms

Being a busy mom can be challenging and time-consuming. Between taking care of the kids, managing the household, and working, it's hard to find time for yourself. However, taking care of yourself is essential, and your beauty routine should be a part of that. Here are some simple beauty routines for busy moms that won't take up too much time.

1. Cleanse, tone, and moisturize

Cleansing, toning, and moisturizing should be the foundation of your beauty routine. It's essential to keep your skin clean and hydrated. Use a gentle cleanser that won't strip your skin of its natural oils. Follow it up with a toner that helps balance your skin's pH and prepare it for moisturizer. Finish with a moisturizer that suits your skin type.

2. Use multitasking products

Using multitasking products can save you time and effort. Look for a tinted moisturizer that provides coverage and hydration. Use a lip and cheek tint that can double as a blush and lip color. You can also use a tinted brow gel that fills in your brows and keeps them in place.

3. Invest in a good dry shampoo

Washing your hair every day can be time-consuming, and it's not suitable for your hair's health. Invest in a good dry shampoo that can refresh your hair between washes. Spray it on your roots, massage it in, and brush it out. Voila! Fresh-looking hair in minutes.

4. Take care of your nails

Taking care of your nails doesn't have to be time-consuming. Keep them trimmed, filed, and clean. Apply a clear or nude polish that doesn't chip easily. If you're feeling fancy, you can use a quick-dry topcoat that saves you time and prevents smudging.

In conclusion, being a busy mom doesn't mean you have to neglect your beauty routine. Follow these simple routines that won't take too much time, and you'll feel confident and radiant in no time. Remember, taking care of yourself is essential, and it's okay to prioritize yourself once in a while.

Tips for involving your children in organic beauty practices

As a young mom or a 30-year-old, you are already aware of the importance of using organic beauty products. But, have you ever thought about involving your children in the same? It's never too early to start teaching your kids about the importance of organic beauty practices. Not only will it instill good habits in them, but it will also help them understand the importance of taking care of their skin and hair from an early age.

Here are some tips for involving your children in organic beauty practices:

1. Start with natural ingredients: Instead of buying chemical-laden beauty products, start by using natural ingredients to make DIY beauty products. Involve your children in the process of making face masks or hair masks using natural ingredients like honey, avocado, or coconut oil. This will not only be fun for them but will also teach them the benefits of using natural ingredients.

2. Teach them about the importance of sunscreen: Sunscreen is essential for protecting the skin from harmful UV rays. Teach your children about the importance of using sunscreen and make sure they wear it every time they step out of the house. You can also buy organic sunscreen for them, which is free from harmful chemicals.

3. Encourage them to drink water: Drinking water is essential for healthy skin and hair. Encourage your children to drink plenty of water throughout the day. You can make it fun by giving them their own water bottle with fun designs or characters.

4. Choose organic beauty products: When buying beauty products for your kids, choose organic and natural products that are free from harmful chemicals. Look for products that are specifically designed for children, such as organic baby lotion or shampoo.

5. Make it fun: Make organic beauty practices fun for your children. You can organize a spa day at home, where you can all pamper yourself with natural beauty products. You can also buy natural and organic makeup for your teenage daughters and teach them how to apply it.

In conclusion, involving your children in organic beauty practices can be a fun and educational experience for both you and your children. By teaching them about the importance of using natural and organic beauty products, you are setting them up for a lifetime of healthy skin and hair.

Conclusion

Recap of the book

Organic Beauty on a Budget: Tips and Tricks for 30 Year Olds is a comprehensive guide for anyone who is looking to embrace natural, organic beauty products while still staying within their budget. This book is perfect for young adults, 30 year olds, and young moms who are interested in organic skincare, natural makeup, and vegan beauty products.

The book is divided into several chapters, each of which provides valuable tips and tricks for anyone who wants to make the switch to organic beauty products. The first chapter provides an introduction to organic beauty and explains why it is important to use natural, organic products on your skin. The chapter also provides tips on how to read product labels and how to identify the ingredients that are harmful to your skin.

The second chapter focuses on organic skincare and provides tips on how to create a skincare routine that is tailored to your skin type. The chapter also provides information on the different types of organic skincare products available in the market and how to choose the right ones for your skin.

The third chapter is all about natural makeup and provides tips on how to create a makeup look that is natural and organic. The chapter also provides information on the different types of natural makeup products available in the market and how to choose the right ones for your skin.

The fourth chapter focuses on vegan beauty products and provides tips on how to identify vegan products and how to incorporate them into your beauty routine. The chapter also provides information on the different types of vegan beauty products available in the market and how to choose the right ones for your skin.

Overall, Organic Beauty on a Budget: Tips and Tricks for 30 Year Olds is a must-read for anyone who is interested in organic skincare, natural makeup, and vegan beauty products. The book provides valuable information on how to make the switch to organic beauty products without breaking the bank, and it is the perfect guide for anyone who wants to embrace a natural, organic lifestyle.

Final thoughts on organic beauty

As we come to the end of this journey through the world of organic beauty, it's important to reflect on what we've learned and how we can apply it to our lives. For young adults, 30 year olds, and young moms, the importance of organic and natural beauty products cannot be overstated. Not only do they offer a safer, healthier alternative to traditional beauty products, but they also provide a more sustainable option for the environment.

When it comes to organic skincare, the key is to focus on ingredients that are natural and gentle on the skin. Look for products that use ingredients like aloe vera, chamomile, and jojoba oil, which can soothe and nourish the skin without causing irritation. And don't forget to protect your skin from the sun's harmful rays with a natural sunscreen.

When it comes to natural makeup, the options are endless. Many brands now offer a wide range of organic and vegan beauty products, including foundation, mascara, and lipstick. These products are often made with ingredients like shea butter and coconut oil, which can help moisturize and protect the skin while providing a flawless finish.

For those who are interested in vegan beauty products, there are many options available as well. These products are made without any animal-derived ingredients and are often cruelty-free as well. Look for products that are certified by organizations like PETA or Leaping Bunny to ensure that they meet these standards.

Overall, the key to incorporating organic and natural beauty products into your routine is to do your research. Look for brands that prioritize sustainability and transparency, and don't be afraid to ask questions about the ingredients used in their products. By making small changes to your beauty routine, you can make a big difference in your health and the health of the planet.

Encouragement to continue practicing organic beauty practices.

Encouragement to continue practicing organic beauty practices

Maintaining a healthy and radiant skin is not always easy, especially with the countless beauty products available in the market today that promise to deliver instant results. However, the truth is that most of these commercial beauty products contain harsh chemicals, synthetic fragrances, and preservatives that can do more harm than good to your skin. This is why it is essential to continue practicing organic beauty practices that are not only safe but also effective.

Organic beauty products are made with natural, plant-based ingredients that are free from harmful chemicals. These products work in harmony with your skin to nourish, protect, and rejuvenate it, leaving you with a healthy, glowing complexion. Unlike commercial beauty products, organic products are gentle on your skin, making them perfect for people with sensitive skin.

Organic skincare is an excellent way to maintain healthy and beautiful skin without breaking the bank. With a few simple steps, you can create an effective organic skincare routine that will keep your skin looking its best. Start by cleansing your skin with a gentle organic cleanser that removes dirt and impurities without stripping your skin of its natural oils. Follow up with an organic toner that balances your skin's pH levels and prepares it for the next steps in your routine.

Next, apply an organic serum that targets your specific skin concerns. Whether you are looking to reduce fine lines, brighten your complexion, or hydrate your skin, there is an organic serum that can help. Finish your routine with an organic moisturizer that locks in moisture and keeps your skin hydrated throughout the day.

When it comes to makeup, natural and vegan beauty products are the way to go. These products are made with natural, plant-based ingredients that are gentle on your skin and the environment. They are free from harsh chemicals, synthetic fragrances, and animal products, making them perfect for people with sensitive skin or those who follow a vegan lifestyle.

Young adults, 30 year olds, and young moms should continue practicing organic beauty practices for many reasons. Firstly, organic products are gentle on your skin, making them perfect for people with sensitive skin. Secondly, they are effective and affordable, making it easy to maintain healthy and beautiful skin without breaking the bank. Lastly, organic beauty practices are better for the environment, making them a great choice for people who are environmentally conscious.

In conclusion, organic beauty practices are a great way to maintain healthy and beautiful skin without compromising your health or the environment. By continuing to use organic beauty products, you can enjoy a radiant complexion that looks and feels great. So, go ahead and start incorporating organic beauty practices into your daily routine. Your skin will thank you for it!

www.ingramcontent.com/pod-product-compliance
Lightning Source LLC
Chambersburg PA
CBHW051851250726
48659CB00006B/2154